Keto Clarity

Ketogenic Diet for
Natural Weight Loss
and Living Healthy Lifestyle

WaraWaran Roongruangsri

Pawana Publishing
Good Health Content

AUTHOR'S NOTE

A diet with low carbohydrate and high fat is called Ketogenic diet. It is the kind of diet which is becoming widely popular these days. There are many benefits of following a ketogenic diet ranging from weight loss to treatment for certain health conditions like neurotic diseases and epilepsy.

Developing a diet that includes low carbohydrate food has been followed by many people to reduce their weight. Ketogenic diet is very helpful for weight loss as it burns the fat in the body, and not carbohydrates. This book includes valuable information on ketogenic diet and the benefits which will follow. It acts as a guide on stepping into ketogenic lifestyle with weekly plan and recipes. Moreover, you can put your own ideas on making food that constitutes low carbohydrate ingredients.

Ketogenic diet would be a good choice for you if you have tried and tested many other dietary programs. The reason for many of dietary failures is that we bother about minimizing the quantity of food and does not think about the content of food. Ketogenic diet helps you to follow a diet program which will include meals of high fat, medium protein and low carbohydrate.

It has been proven scientifically that ketogenic diet program is very effective for weight loss. You get to eat every food you love, but limiting on the quantity in a better way that you are used to do. You need not have to stay hungry as part of dieting when you follow ketogenic way of diet program. It works well for your stomach and body as well.

You can download the book "Keto Clarity: Ketogenic Diet for Natural Weight Loss and Living Healthy Lifestyle" for better awareness on the health benefits of ketogenic diet.

This book includes valuable information on ketogenic diets, the different benefits you get from it, the ways to switch into ketogenic diet program, pros and cons of this diet program from experienced dieticians, the types of food you should eat, along with some other helpful tips.

Through this book, we look forward to making you informed about improving your health and body metabolism, while staying fit. We welcome you to the innovative dietary program, which is effective and perhaps the best for burning the fat.

This book includes the following chapters:
- Keto Clarity: Ketogenic Dieting Made Easy
- Ketogenic Diets and Their Rapid Weight Loss Effects
- Ketosis - The Cyclical Ketogenic Diet Fat Burn
- The Benefits of Ketogenic Diet in Weight Loss System
- Ketogenic Diet Plan - The Best Fat Burning Diet
- Why Did I Choose a Ketogenic Lifestyle? Review
- Much, much more!

Thanks for downloading the book. I am sure you will enjoy reading it!

WaraWaran Roongruangsri.

CONTENTS

1. KETO CLARITY: KETOGENIC DIETING MADE EASY

It has been believed that in order to lose your weight, you have to limit your fat intake. These days the notion is changing as there are research papers coming out which stick to the fact that you can reduce fat faster by limiting the intake of carbohydrate foods, and by increasing the quantity of fatty foods.

Sources of energy for the body

Generally, body absorbs energy from carbohydrates, then fat and also from proteins, if necessary, for its daily activities. Imagine the condition when body gets low carbohydrate. It will automatically go after the fat content, which is another source of fuel. However, the body has the ability to manufacture carbohydrates by a reaction between protein and glycerol, which is a component of fat.

What are ketones?

The fat content in the body is used as secondary fuel source by all parts of the body other than brain and the nervous system. Ketones make the fuel source for brains and nervous system. The fact is that all parts of nervous system can function quite well even without carbohydrates, as ketones make their primary source of fuel. Now what are ketones? It is a bye product formed after the incomplete breakdown of fatty acids in the liver.

Suppose you are on a ketogenic diet for a period of time. The body will switch to a condition in which more ketones will be manufactured. Subsequently, the conversion of protein to energy will be limited. The body will burn more calories to keep lean body mass or muscle. This is one of the primary reasons for the ketogenic diet to be more effective.

How body accepts to ketogenic diet ?

Normally, body takes about twenty one days to adjust to consumption of fatty acids and ketones as energy source. The body takes its own time to switch to the new source of energy, as it is used to carbohydrates for long. Suddenly when you limit the carbohydrate intake to zero, the body will definitely take some time to adjust to it. It has to be noted that obviously you will feel tired for the first few days once you start on a ketogenic diet. You may feel difficult to concentrate, may feel nauseated etc. But be sure, once your body accepts the new source of fuel, it will do wonders on you.

Insulin and glucagon are two hormones which are mostly affected once you get into a diet that includes low carbohydrate and high fat foods. Insulin is the transporting agent of nutrients from blood to cells. On the other hand, glucagon is responsible for cells to release nutrients to the blood stream. There will be search for an alternate source of glucose, when the normal source is limited.

In the ketogenic diet, the body will produce more glucagon and less insulin. The carbohydrates in the blood stream start to release the fat deposits. It will be metabolized. As a result, ketone production will increase and body will reach a situation called ketosis.

How to attain Ketosis ?

Ketogenic diet is mainly stick on the concept of low carbohydrate diet and there are many ways to reach the condition of ketosis. Here go few types of ketogenic diet and helpful information on following it including training plans.

The maximum and minimum intake of carbohydrate depends on each individual. However, carbohydrate at the level of 30-50gm with higher intake of fatty foods and 1-2 g of protein per kg is recommended.

Benefits of ketogenic diet

There are many benefits of following a ketogenic diet. Check out the list.

- A good thing about ketogenic is that you don't feel hungry even when you are on a diet program for it controls appetite.
- The fat loss will be more efficient and fast than other methods.
- The muscle loss will remain minimal, but you may feel your strength becoming low.
- Ketones keep you in good mood always.
- You will be able to have a dietary meal, that too with happy mind.

WaraWaran Roongruangsri

2. KETOGENIC DIETS AND THEIR RAPID WEIGHT LOSS EFFECTS

On a general note, all dietary programs for weight loss focus on calorie reduction or limiting the intake of proteins, fats or carbohydrates, which are essential nutrients of the body.

Ketogenic dietary program was first put forward by Johns Hopkins Pediatric Epilepsy Center and Dr R.M. Wilder of the Mayo Clinic in the early 1920's. Actually, the diets were designed to copy the biochemical changes happening with fasting, acidosis and dehydration. The diet primarily constituted 10-15 grams of carbohydrates in a day with 1 gram of protein per kilogram bodyweight of the individual and rest from fats.

The word meaning of ketogenic is nothing but increasing the production of ketones in body and this will cause higher lipolysis or breaking down of fat in common terms. The equation of ketogenic diet equals high fat, moderate protein and high protein, moderate fat, but minimal carbohydrate. As we told in the beginning, ketones are the acidic by-products while liver breaks down fat into fatty acids.

According to the supporters of ketogenic diet, people gain weight because of high glycamic index, a component of carbohydrate. Usually carbohydrate breaks itself into glucose, a form of sugar which is a source of energy. Although the body has the ability to break glycogen and fat and use it as a source of energy, but it normally chooses the other way. That makes carbohydrates the major cause of weight gain.

Over production of insulin occurs with higher intake of glycemic index carbohydrate foods, and it is where the weight gain starts. Insulin is responsible for regulating blood glucose level and in turn it controls the weight by managing the energy equation of the body. Increased glucose content in the bloodstream will lead to excessive secretion of insulin. The excess glucose will be stored as glycogen or as fatty acids.

For that reason, Ketogenic diet aims at controlling insulin production to its lowest range by significantly reducing the carbohydrate consumption. The body will be provided with fatty foods and protein rich foods as source of energy.

However, the main aim of ketogenic diets is to help the body to attain the state of ketosis. Wondering what will be the mechanism in ketosis state? Well, ketosis is a condition in which rate of ketone production is higher than the ability of tissues to oxidize it. Earlier it was mentioned how ketone is produced in the body. Ketosis is actually a side effect that happens if you take low carbohydrate foods, and it is a secondary product of lipolysis. And definitely Ketogenic diets encourage ketosis.

The state of ketosis is usually attained when you stay hungry for long time. Ketosis can also be induced by a diet that includes low carbohydrate or low calorie food with higher quantities of fats or proteins. In fact, high fat and high protein diets are inducing the state of ketosis intentionally.

You might have understood by now that ketosis is another efficient way of energy production by burning the fat deposits, rather than by producing insulin. In low carbohydrate consumption, body reduces insulin production and burns the fats instead. So eventually it is one the best possible ways to reduce the body weight in a short span of time.

Ketogenic diets are formulated to initially force the body to exhaust its glucose supply and then switch to fat burning process. Later, once the state of ketosis is attained, food supply is meant to keep the fat burning process running by adjusting further consumption of carbohydrates and give the body minimum amount of calories needed.

Take the example of Atkins diet, which is probably the most attractive diet program. It helps individuals to attain the diet program which is called Critical Carbohydrate Level for Maintenance abbreviated as CCLM. In Atkins diet, the dieter neither gains nor loses weight.

It was in 2003 that a modified version of Atkins diet was developed by John Hopkins treatment centre. It was actually formulated to treat 20 children who were suffering from epilepsy. The treatment showed the results that said two thirds of the children had significantly reduced their seizures. While nine of them could reduce the medicine intake, none of them developed kidney stones.

Apart from that, there are continuing studies on the effects of ketogenic diet by National Institute of Health (NIH). Moreover, better versions of Atkins diet are being developed which helps people to lose weight and treat epilepsy.

Interestingly, National Institute of Neurological Disorders and Stroke (NINDS) is also researching on effects of ketogenic diets and also on medications for weight reduction.

Keto Clarity

3. KETOSIS - THE CYCLICAL KETOGENIC DIET FAT BURN

We would like to make you more informed by giving you a clear picture about cyclical ketogenic diet. This chapter will describe the reactions that happen in your body while starting with ketogenic diet.

In the state of ketosis, body becomes an autopilot for burning fat. The fat deposits in your body get used as energy source and this causes the reduction of weight. But it does not affect the water or muscle in the body.

Most of the diet programs encourage food with low calorie. The weight loss in those diet programs normally causes weight reduction in the form of water and muscle, with low importance to fats deposits. The metabolism of the body gets slower as body gets the notion that you are starving and so have to reduce the process of losing calories. Slow metabolism will lead to slower weight loss and faster weight gain.

In ketogenic diets, it is about carbohydrate reduction. It is to restrict carbohydrate and maintain calories, so that there will be no option left for the body for energy source other than burning the fats. In fact, ketosis is such a condition in which you switch on your fat burning machine naturally.

Ketones are excreted from your body by the key player and the largest internal organ, liver. The liver is responsible for converting fat into ketones. Both the fatty acids are broken and ketones are created in the liver. But ketones will be formed only when there is lack of sugar and glucose in the body. You know carbohydrate includes sugar and glucose and it makes tough to reduce weight when you are in a high carbohydrate diet. In a ketogenic diet, we reduce both glucose and sugar, and the body will have to burn fat and thus produces ketones.

Naturally, the ketones are sent out of the body which is other ways fat loss and in turn weight reduction.

There are many myths surrounding the ketogenic diet and we want you to belief the facts. Our body can obviously be healthy in ketosis on a long term. On a further note, the ketosis is very much natural when sugar and glucose level is minimized. And it is absolutely normal for the body to act this way. In simple words, it is safe to burn fat!

Imagine now you are on a ketogenic diet but confused whether the body is burning the fat deposits. You can make sure that your body is burning the fat by using a ketone testing strips, which is easily available at the pharmacist. You can capture few drops of urine on the strip and look for a change in color. Pink to purple means a favorable result. You will be able to know whether the body is in a fat burning zone by checking the color scale.

These strips will be in handy for you to realize the release of ketones. By this way, you can know whether you are keeping the carbohydrate intake at its minimum level. Even if you are not getting the dark purple in the strip, it is not a matter of worry as each individual's body responds at different levels. Moreover, you are perfectly alright if you are losing weight while on your ketogenic diet.

In ketogenic diet, you have to check the water intake is sufficient. In case if the strip is showing dark purple every day, you need to be conscious. It may be a sign of dehydration, which means you need to increase the water intake.

Remember that your fat burning mechanism is switched on with the cyclical ketogenic diet. You are restricting the carbohydrate intake and tempting the body to burn the fat reserves for weight loss. Check the level of fat being burned with the help of ketone strips.

Keto Clarity

4. THE BENEFITS YOU OF KETOGENIC DIET IN WEIGHT LOSS SYSTEM

Ketogenic diet weight programs are indeed one of the most discussed ways of weight loss these days and works effectively for many people. Diets with extremely low carbohydrate diets will take you to a state of ketosis and this burn the fatty reserves in your body. The state of ketosis is achieved by depriving the body of glucose. The food source is available through a nutritional diet plan.

Here are few benefits of ketogenic diet program that you might be interested to know

1.   Perhaps the state of ketosis is the best way to make the body use fat as a energy fuel. Actually, it is easier for body to use carbohydrates as a fuel. When your carbohydrate intake is high, the body will concentrate more on burning it, and does not bother about the fat reserves.

2.   It is a natural fact that ketones are no way

harmful for the body system on any grounds. The excess ketones are simply excreted by your body though urine, without being harmful or worrisome. Furthermore, you get to check the amount of fat burning in your body by an easy ketone strip test.

3.   Once your body is in ketosis state, it will prefer ketones to glucose. Your body does not crave for sugar now, and will accept protein as a good source of fuel.

4.   Next benefit is that your insulin levels will be controlled on a ketogenic diet. As you know, insulin is a prominent factor for weight gain as you crave for more sugary foods.

5.   People often reviews that they do not feel hungry when they are on kretogenic diet format compared to other diet programs. It is very much easier to start with a diet, but the craving and the huger would tempt you to break it in the middle. Obviously, the result of the diet will be disappointing. In ketogenic diet, you don't feel hungry and so the probability of diet plan success is higher. It makes easier for you to reach your weight loss goals in a much easier way.

I hope you are now better informed about the ketogenic weight loss plan. You may be more attracted towards this weight loss plan. You can give a try on this diet program as you are not going to lose anything else other than weight.

5. KETOGENIC DIET PLAN – THE BEST FAT BURNING DIET

If you want to rapidly reduce the weight and burn the fat using natural ways, then ketogenic diet is the most apt one for you. You do not need to over exercise, if you are on a state of ketosis.

What is a ketogenic diet plan?

Ketogenic diet plan simply helps body to enter into the state of ketosis. It is pretty much natural and healthy metabolic way of body burning the reserved body fat and thereby promoting the creation of ketones, instead of glucose. Glucose is the sugars from carbohydrates that make a component for Standard American Diet abbreviated as SAD.

Ketogenic way is powerful and contains food that increases metabolism. Moreover, ketogenic plan includes delicious and natural foods, that is healthy as well as tasteful.

The foods that needs to be encouraged
Well, ketogenic plan includes some tasteful and delicious food, like beef and chicken, healthy sources of protein, and high quality fatty foods like eggs, butter, olive oil, coconut oil and avocado. Leafy vegetables like kale, chard, spinach and cruciferous vegetables like broccoli, cabbage and cauliflower. Added to it are seeds, nuts, sprouts, and also many other wonderful food items. This diet gives you amazing health benefits while providing the body with essential protein, fats and nutrients. Furthermore, the metabolism boosting meals are easy to cook at home and also effortlessly available if you are on a travel.

The food that needs to be limited
The foods that need to be avoided in ketogenic plan include everything that has high carbohydrates, sugar and also fatty foods that is bad for health. Intake of these foods increases the level of insulin and blood sugar in the body and the fat gets stored as a result. Such foods can turn toxic for the body by creating excess glucose levels. In order to avoid these components, stay away from eating grains, processed foods, vegetable oils made of canola, corn and soybean, milk, margarine, and many other high-carbohydrate and high sugar foods.

Are n't fatty foods bad?
There is a common belief that in order to reduce weight, you need to limit fatty foods. This theory is widely encouraged by government institutions as well as industrial organizations. However, the modern understanding of human nutrition is against these beliefs. Factually, certain fats are not good for health, like omega-6 fatty acids, since your body has hard time processing them. Some other fats like triglycerides are particularly beneficial for losing weight, brain cell generation and nutrient supply. The healthy saturated fats have to be encouraged while the detrimental trans-fat should be limited to minimum. It is

usually found in processed foods.

The benefits of ketogenic diet plan
Here go the benefits of following ketogenic diet plan.

It burns stored fat

A ketogenic diet plan encourages the body to consume the stored fat in the body and creates ketone by breaking down fatty acids. As said earlier, it lowers the glucose production caused by higher level of carbohydrates in diet. The ketones do the job of glucose. This in turn will result in rapid reduction of fats.

It retains muscle mass

In a ketogenic diet, the right fats are induced in your food. The existing fat deposits become the source of energy by getting converted into useful sugars and ketones. Furthermore, this will be an essential source of energy for the brain, muscles and heart. The major benefit in this process rests in preserving muscle mass, as the body does not need to tap into muscle protein. So the benefit of ketogenic diet is double as it retains muscle mass and reduces body weight.

It eliminates excess fat

The unwanted body fat will be excreted out in ketogenic diet program. The reserved fat in the body are converted into ketones and there will be over production of ketones. But it will not do any harm to the body as it gets out of the system through urine.

It reduces appetite

As the ketogenic diet plan regulates the powerful

metabolic hormones in the body, the appetite will be consistently controlled. It lowers the insulin production and promotes the creation of ketones. As you know the low calorie carbohydrate rich food will make you hungrier often. You will not feel hungry on this diet and it is one of the best advantages of this diet plan.

So what more to wait? Start your weight loss plan by burning the fat and not by over exercising! You can control the metabolism of the body naturally by adopting to a ketogenic diet plan. Realize the fact that your body is best suited for this style of nutrition.

The metabolic state of the body can be optimized by taking delicious foods that our ancient generation followed. It never included carbohydrate-rich processed foods loaded with sugars and bad fats. In this diet, it includes luxurious and fulfilling food items that are inspired by the olden ages. It has lean meat, vegetables, nuts and seeds, and healthy fats that would tickle your taste buds.

WaraWaran Roongruangsri

6. WHY DID I CHOOSE A KETOGENIC LIFESTYLE? A REVIEW

When I entered into ketogenic diet plan, my primary goal was to shed extra pounds. I call myself a 'recovering fatass' like the way that someone who quit alcohol would be called as 'recovering alcohol.' I have a history of struggling with body weight all my life and I had less hope of meeting my goals after experimenting on variety of diet plans.

I was attracted towards ketogenic diet as it limits carbohydrate intake and burn the stored fats and thereby I can lose my weight. But to my surprise, I got additional control of my body with this new form of diet. That made me happy as I'm interested in life-hacking and "mind over matter."

Moreover, I was inclined towards ketogenic diet as it reduces my appetite, but keep me healthy. It is a fact that if you are on a diet, the hungry feel is so awful to manage. Often we can't resist the temptation to eat those foods which we crave for.

Most people on ketogenic diet share their experience that after eating a ketogenic diet for two weeks, they do not feel hungry like before, even on a calorie-reduced diet! It lessens the chance of missing the diet plan as you do not feel hungry.

I am fascinated by this diet plan as I get to eat foods that I like even when I am on it. I am a foodie and I love cooking too. It is unbelievable that I could find a diet plan where I can include fatty foods as I please. However, this is not a diet plan that suggests you can eat whatever you fancy, and in whichever quantity.

Losing weight is, in essence, math... if you eat in fewer calories than you expend, you can expect to drop weight, full stop. But by making the calories I'm taking in delicious, I won't crave extras, and I'm going to be more likely to follow my plan. Or at the least this is the theory.

That was all about my fascination towards a ketogenic diet program. We will go in detail about the science behind the ketogenic diet on another book. At least right now you know what got me moving on my fat-burning journey.

Keto Clarity

7. CONCLUSION

As per expert opinion, ketongenic is a rapid way to lose weight. It provides the principles of maintaining a healthy shape for long term. Although Ketogenic diet was originally created for medical purposes to treat epilepsy in children, soon it was identified as an effective weight loss plan.

It is a misguiding fact that fat is unhealthy. On the contrary, 'good' fats are essential to a nutritious diet. The goal of ketogenic diet is to make body accept its energy source as fats, instead of carbohydrates. The body will be attained to a state of ketosis in few days and result will be rapid weight loss. The ketogenic diet is high in fat, low in carbohydrates, and is designed to provide adequate protein and calories for a healthy weight.

In ketogenic diet, you exclude high carbohydrate foods like starchy fruits, vegetables, bread, pasta and sugar. On the other hand, you increase the intake of fatty foods like cream and butter. Say for a typical meal, it will be fish or chicken with green vegetables and fruit with lots of cream. Your breakfast may include bacon or eggs, a snack cheese with cucumber.

Ketogenic diet is not only a weight loss program, but also makes a healthier life style. You will have long lasting benefits of staying fit and slim in this diet. The success factor behind this diet plan is you do not feel hungry often and so higher chances of meeting the goal of weigh reduction.

People who have practiced ketogenic diets often review as they have increased energy levels. In short, the ketogenic plan improves the quality of life in every way.

Finally, if you have enjoyed this book, shall I ask for a favor? Will you be kind enough to leave a review for this book on Amazon? Well, It'd be greatly appreciated!

Thank you and good luck!

WaraWaran Roongruangsri.

ABOUT THE AUTHOR

WaraWaran Roongruangsri is a highly accomplished food specialist, university instructor, and nutritionist. She is best known for her expertise in food nutrition, healthy living and natural diet that allow the modern woman to lead a more well balanced lifestyle.

As the nutrition and health expert, WaraWaran shares reliable, practical, and easy to follow advice that helps people eat better, live healthier, and lead more fulfilling lives.

WaraWaran lives in Chiangmai Thailand, currently working as a university lecturer and also work as nutritionist base on academic research career. She believes that it's never too early to start and it's never too late to make a healthy lifestyle.

A wise man once said...
To eat is a necessity, but to eat intelligently is an art
- Francois de la Rochefoucauld